Unlocking the Secrets of Science

Profiling 20th Century Achievers in Science, Medicine, and Technology

Willem Kolff and the Invention of the Dialysis Machine

Kathleen Tracy

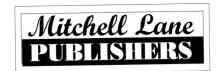

Mitchell Lane
PUBLISHERS

PO Box 619 • Bear, Delaware 19701
www.mitchelllane.com

Unlocking the Secrets of Science

Profiling 20th Century Achievers in Science, Medicine, and Technology

Willem Kolff and the Invention of the Dialysis Machine

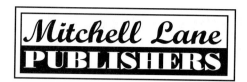

Printing   1   2   3   4   5   6   7   8   9   10

Library of Congress Cataloging-in-Publication Data

Tracy, Kathleen.
     Willem Kolff and the invention of the dialysis machine/Kathleen Tracy
        p. cm. — (Unlocking the secrets of science)
     Summary: A biography of the Dutch doctor who worked to perfect a means of treating kidney failure and later helped develop the first artificial heart.
     Includes bibliographical references and index.
     ISBN 1-58415-135-8 (lib. bdg.)
     1. Kolff, Willem J., 1912—Juvenile literature. 2. Hemodialysis—History—Juvenile literature. 3. Artificial kidney—History—Juvenile literature. 4. Physicians—Netherlands—Biography—Juvenile literature. [1. Kolff, Willem J., 1912- 2. Physicians. 3. Artificial kidney—History.] I. Title. II. Series.
RC901.7.H45 K658 2002
617.4'61059'092—dc21
[B]
                                              2002066126

ABOUT THE AUTHOR: Kathleen Tracy has been a journalist for over twenty years. Her writing has been featured in magazines including The Toronto Star's "Star Week," *A&E Biography* magazine, *KidScreen* and *TV Times*. She is also the author of numerous biographies including "The Boy Who Would Be King" (Dutton), "Jerry Seinfeld - The Entire Domain" (Carol Publishing) and "Don Imus - America's Cowboy" (Carroll & Graf). She recently completed "God's Will?" for Sourcebooks.

CHILDREN'S SCIENCE REVIEW EDITOR: Stephanie Kondrchek, B.S. Microbiology, University of Maryland

PHOTO CREDITS: cover: Hank Morgan/Photo Researchers; p. 10 AP Photo; p. 12 Hank Morgan/Photo Researchers; p. 18 Corbis; p. 30 Corbis; p. 33 Hank Morgan/ Photo Researchers; pp. 36, 38, 39, 40 Corbis.

PUBLISHER'S NOTE: In selecting those persons to be profiled in this series, we first attempted to identify the most notable accomplishments of the 20th century in science, medicine, and technology. When we were done, we noted a serious deficiency in the inclusion of women. For the greater part of the 20th century science, medicine, and technology were male-dominated fields. In many cases, the contributions of women went unrecognized. Women have tried for years to be included in these areas, and in many cases, women worked side by side with men who took credit for their ideas and discoveries. Even as we move forward into the 21st century, we find women still sadly underrepresented. It is not an oversight, therefore, that we profiled mostly male achievers. Information simply does not exist to include a fair selection of women.

Contents

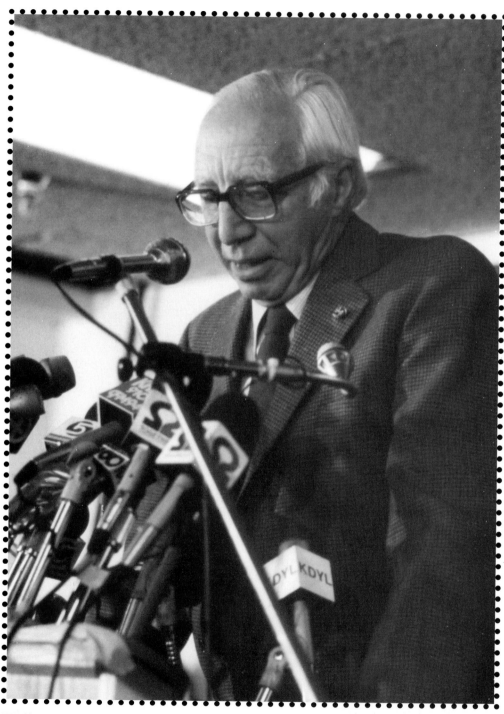

Willem Kolff, a pioneer in the development of the artificial heart and kidney, is shown here talking to the media.

Chapter 1

A Patient Named Jan

• •

Europe in 1938 was an uneasy place. Adolf Hitler's Nazi party had risen to power in Germany, and neighboring countries watched with concern as the German military grew in strength and size. It was amid these winds of war that young Willem Kolff graduated with a medical degree from the University of Leyden in The Netherlands, a country that is sometimes also called Holland.

Although he was technically no longer a student, Kolff was an idealistic and intensely curious young doctor who was eager to keep learning. In October 1938 he accepted a nonpaying job at the University of Groningen Hospital as an assistant in the Department of Medicine. He was made responsible for four beds. If only one bed was occupied, then he only had one patient to take care of; if all four were filled, then he had to look after all four patients.

Occupying one of the beds was a patient named Jan Bruning. Jan was only 22 years old and had been admitted to the hospital suffering from a kidney disease called glomerulonephritis, in which the capillaries, or small blood vessels, in the kidney are inflamed. Jan's condition was chronic, meaning he had been afflicted with the disease a long time. The disease had finally caused his kidneys to stop filtering toxic waste products out of Jan's blood. As these waste products accumulated in his body, Jan was slowly being poisoned to death, a condition called uremia.

The kidneys are a pair of bean-shaped organs, about the size of an adult fist, located in the lower back on either side

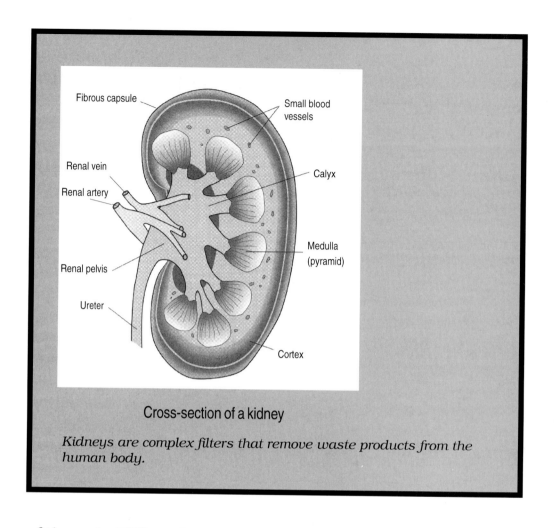

Cross-section of a kidney

Kidneys are complex filters that remove waste products from the human body.

of the spine. They do several very important jobs. First, they remove waste products and excess fluid from the body via urine. Second, they keep a number of minerals in proper balance, including salt and potassium. They also produce a hormone called erythropoietin that plays a part in the production of red blood cells; these blood cells carry oxygen throughout the body. Without the work of the kidneys, a person will die. Jan Bruning's kidneys were failing.

Even for a doctor, watching someone die of kidney failure, or end-stage renal disease, is agonizing. The symptoms of uremia cause patients much suffering and include nausea, headache, dizziness, dry skin and rapid pulse. As the fluids and waste products were building up in Jan's body, he suffered from edema, swelling of the hands and feet. Hypertension caused his skin to look red and flushed. His eyesight failed and his breath smelled of urine. And as the concentration of urea—the waste product created when the body breaks down protein—increased, it began to crystallize through his skin, causing unbearable itching. Jan couldn't even enjoy a meal: he vomited any food he tried to eat.

On the last Sunday in October 1938, Jan's mother came to the hospital to see her son. She had dressed up for the occasion, wearing a beautiful silk dress and a lace cap she had sewn herself. However, Jan could not see it because he had gone blind.

In an interview conducted by the American Academy of Achievement, Kolff recalled how Bruning "slowly and miserably died from renal failure. And I, as a very, very young physician, had to tell his mother, in a black dress and a little white cap like the farm women have, that her only son was going to die. I couldn't do a damn thing about it."

Three days after his mother's visit, Jan went into a coma; the day after that he died. Kolff was deeply affected, but rather than let the feeling of helplessness defeat him, he thought about how Jan's death could have been prevented. "I began to think, *If I could just every day remove as much urea as this boy creates, which is about 20 grams, then the boy could live.*" Although he knew what would have saved his patient, Kolff did not have a way to accomplish it. He did not know how to get the urea out of a person's body. So, he recalled, "I began to work on that."

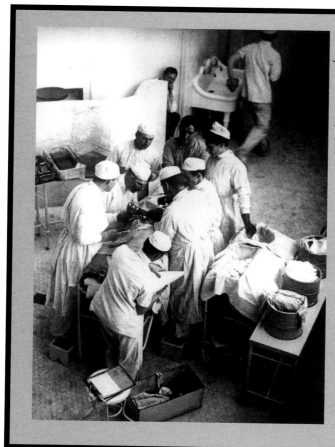

When Kolff graduated from medical school in 1938, surgery was still in its infancy. This photo shows a surgical procedure at Johns Hopkins Hospital in the early 1900s.

Kolff began reading every book he could find in the university's library on purifying the blood. He discovered that other doctors had tried to solve the same problem. Animal research conducted two decades earlier had shown that it was possible to dialyze, or remove the toxins from, the blood using special membranes, then return the blood to the animal's body. The first practical demonstration of this process, known as continuous dialysis of blood, was made in 1913 by the American research team of John Jacob Abel, Leonard Rowntree and J.J. Turner at Johns Hopkins Hospital in Baltimore. The team called the process vividiffusion.

The doctors used rabbits and dogs for their experiments. After two to three hours of dialysis, the animals made complete recoveries. Although the primary goal of the experiment was to develop a way to measure the concentration of substances such as hormones in the blood, Abel saw greater potential in the process, which is why they called their dialyzer, or dialysis machine, an artificial kidney.

In 1924 German scientist George Haas performed dialysis on the first human patient. He used a process called hemodialysis, which is when a machine of some sort is used to clean wastes from the blood. However, there was still no successful method of filtering the deadly urea out of a patient's body. Moreover, most physicians saw dialysis as simply a temporary treatment for acute renal failure, which is when the kidneys are suddenly but temporarily affected. In those cases, dialysis would keep the patient alive long enough for their kidneys to recover and begin working again.

While that was fine for medical conditions where it was possible to heal the kidney, for people like Jan Bruning, whose kidneys would never work again, it still meant they would die. Kolff looked beyond the thinking of the time and envisioned a kind of dialysis that wouldn't simply be a temporary measure, but would actually take the place of the kidneys and allow people to go on living.

Ironically, in 1913, when Kolff was just two years old, Abel, Rowntree and Turner first presented the results of their research on the artificial kidney at a medical conference held in Groningen—the same Netherlands city where Kolff would later earn his Ph.D. and where, 26 years after the American researchers introduced vividiffusion, he would begin working on a way to conquer kidney failure.

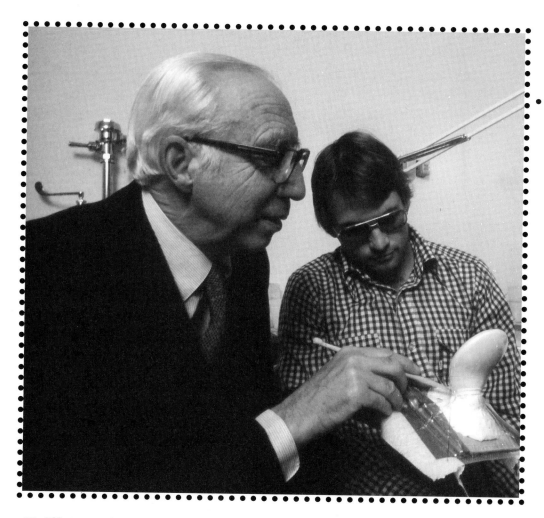

Kolff was also a pioneer in developing artificial limbs. Early in his life, however, he thought he would like to run a zoo. When his father pointed out that there were only three zoos in the Netherlands, Kolff turned his attention elsewhere. But he always had a passion for animals.

Chapter 2

A Reluctant Student

W illem Kolff was born on February 14, 1911. Growing up in Leyden, Holland, he displayed the innate curiosity that would later lead to so many medical discoveries. But even though his father, Jacob, was a physician and the director of a tuberculosis sanatorium, Willem couldn't decide what profession he wanted to pursue. To him, everything sounded interesting. If he had any particular passion as a boy, it was for animals; his pets included rabbits, pigeons, sheep, guinea pigs and pheasants.

Kolff recalled to the American Academy of Achievement, "When I was very young I wanted to become the director of a zoo. But my father pointed out that at that time there were only three zoos in the Netherlands. So your chances of becoming a zoo director were pretty small."

In the Netherlands, children went to school five and a half days a week, including Saturday mornings. After Willem got out of school on the weekends, he had to take carpentry lessons. Jacob wanted his son to at least have a skill that could turn into a career, because although Willem was popular and had a lot of friends, he wasn't the most diligent of students. "No," he admitted, "I was never very good in school. I had a lot of other interests than school."

High school was especially difficult for Willem. "You had to learn four modern languages and you also had to take six years of Latin and five years of Greek," he recalled. "You didn't have electives, you had to take *everything*." As a result of the difficult curriculum, Kolff calls his high school years "perhaps the most difficult of my life. I was forced to do things that I did not really like to do, but I knew that it was necessary," because if you made it through high school, "then any university would be open to you."

What made Willem's homework even more difficult was that he suffered from dyslexia, a learning disorder that makes it hard to read and, in Willem's case, spell. "This plagued me a great deal," he told the Academy. "I like to read, but I read slowly." In the 1920s, dyslexia wasn't well understood, so children who had it were often ridiculed, even by teachers. But Kolff says he simply "learned to live with it. You can overcome it to a great extent by reading and by writing." Although Kolff says he isn't one to give advice, he does encourage all students to keep studying, no matter how hard it is, because to be successful, "you must have an education." However, Kolff also believes, "The guys with very high grades are not necessarily the people that are the most successful in later life," and anyone who works hard "has a chance."

For seven years Kolff learned how to work with wood. He never showed any interest in following in Jacob's footsteps. Part of his aversion to a medical career was seeing how his father anguished over his patients' suffering. Jacob was so dedicated, he would frequently go back to the sanatorium late at night to look after his patients, many of whom were beyond help. "At that time there were no antibiotics and tuberculosis was a terrible disease," Willem Kolff explained.

Willem and his father would take walks though the nearby woods where Jacob "would discuss his worries about his patients. And from him I certainly inherited this extreme concern about the well-being of patients." When patients got better, Jacob would be elated, but, Willem recalled, "I've also seen him crying and desperate after trying for a long time and a patient did not get well, and went home to die." And that was the part of medicine Willem didn't think he could bear. "I didn't want to become a doctor because I didn't want to see people die."

For a long time it seemed that Willem Kolff would be giving his talents to making cabinets as opposed to helping the sick. Eventually, however, Jacob convinced his son to give medicine a chance. Perhaps it was Willem's dread at the thought of watching people die that led him to try to invent machines that would ease pain and prolong life. Although Willem says he never thought of himself becoming an inventor, he admits, "I always wanted to make something."

Willem attended medical school at the well-regarded University of Leyden. Founded in 1575, it's the oldest college in the Netherlands; the city itself dates back to the Roman Empire. At the university, one teacher in particular had a great influence on him. Kolff told the Academy, "During my studies, I became an Assistant in Pathological Anatomy. That old professor, whose name was Tenderloo, was a very scientific man. From him I think I learned the power of reasoning, to be critical about what you think and not assume something that may not be true and that is not proven."

Life at Leyden was quite comfortable for Kolff. He belonged to the student club and says, "I had a man who came in the morning to wake me up and polish my shoes. You lived far above your means. But at that time that was the thing to do."

When Kolff graduated in 1938, he took the job at the University of Groningen Hospital, where he met Jan Bruning. One reason he accepted a nonpaying position was that it was one of the few places that allowed residents to be married. Kolff's wife, Janke, supported them during this time. They lived in a small house while Willem served his residency under Professor Polak Daniels. Daniels was another great influence, because he supported Kolff's dream of developing an artificial kidney.

"There are some professors who want their students to do exactly what the professor is interested in," Kolff noted during his interview with the Academy. "This man was different. He set us free, and when I wanted to pursue a certain thing, he would study it and help." It was a lesson Kolff would remember as he started working with students.

Several years later, after World War II, Willem went back to school at the University of Groningen. He earned a Ph.D. summa cum laude in 1946. But as soon as he qualified for his certificate as a specialist in internal medicine, he decided to leave the hospital for a position in the small town of Kampen.

The reason Kolff left was simple. On May 10, 1940, Germany invaded the Netherlands. Five days later, Holland surrendered and was under complete control of the Nazis. Professor Daniels and his wife, who were Jewish, committed suicide, choosing death over living under Hitler's rule. The effect on Willem was profound. Years later, he would write in the *Annals of Internal Medicine,* "Whereas other members of the staff had shown marked impatience regarding my plans for an artificial kidney, Polak Daniels had allowed me to go ahead without ridiculing the idea. His death left a vacancy."

A short time later, the Germans put a Nazi in Professor Daniels' old position. Kolff refused to work beside any follower of Hitler. However, he said leaving meant "I had to look for a place, and I found one in Kampen. It was a very small hospital. They were very nice to me. They wanted to have an internist, and I was the first. I made the royal sum of 10,000 guilders per year in the first year," the equivalent now of $4,000. With that money, Willem set out to make an artificial kidney.

Kolff began researching in earnest once he was settled in Kampen. His coworkers there remember the young doctor as being tireless and spending a great deal of time with his patients. He also suggested inventive and radical ideas on how to treat them.

But Kolff did more than just imagine. As Hitler continued to plunge Europe into war, destruction and darkness, Willem Kolff set out to create a machine that would save countless lives.

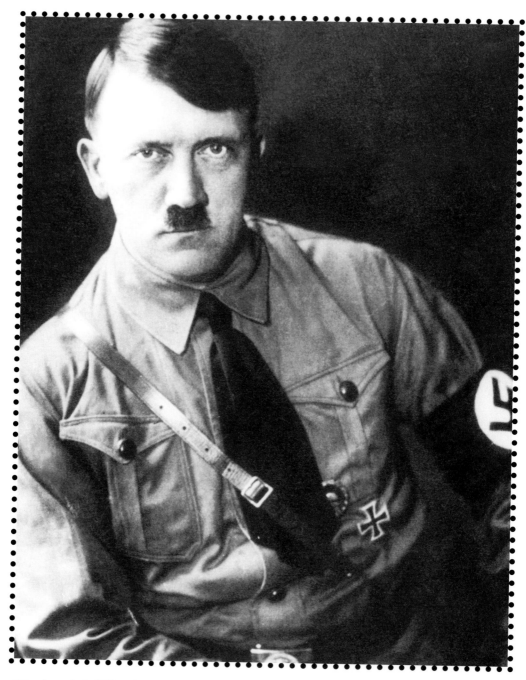

Under Adolf Hitler's rule, the Nazis invaded Holland. But the war could not curb Kolff's inventive mind. Helping the wounded during the war gave Kolff valuable experience he would later use in developing his artificial kidney.

Chapter 3
A Change of Plans

• •

Had war not broken out, Kolff might never have continued his work creating an artificial kidney. During his interview with the American Academy of Achievement, Kolff said that he had originally planned to go to Indonesia to practice medicine.

"Indonesia at that time was a Dutch colony," he explained. "I knew a young doctor could go be the head of the Department of Medicine of a large plantation way in the hinterland, and get wonderful experience. You could be independent, and do very much what you wanted, and still help people. That is what I had planned to do. I even followed a course in tropical medicine, but then the war came, and you couldn't get out."

However, the war could not curb Kolff's inventive mind. In the spring of 1940, when Willem and Janke were in the Netherlands city The Hague for her father's funeral, Germany began its invasion. The Germans sent planes to buzz the Dutch countryside, throwing out fliers warning the people to surrender or else. They also bombed the local army barracks. Willem climbed onto a rooftop to watch the Dutch troops fire back at the German planes, and, typically, his thoughts were on the people who might be injured during the battle.

So while Janke attended her father's funeral, Willem excused himself and went to the local hospital. It had occurred to him that with the onset of war there would soon be a desperate need for blood in order to treat the wounded. Kolff had first gotten interested in blood transfusions while he was working at Groningen. Back in the 1930s, blood was transfused directly from one person to another, with the two people lying side by side. But Kolff used the method we use today of having blood stored in a bag dripped into the patient. "I was the first in the Netherlands—and probably on the continent of Europe—to apply blood by continuous drip," acknowledged Kolff. Although he was quick to point out, "It was not my invention; it was done first in England."

To use that method, there needed to be a way to store the blood. Willem read constantly and came across an article about a blood bank in Chicago, Illinois. Inspired, he dreamed of setting up a similar blood bank in Europe one day. Watching the Germans attacking his country made him think of that blood bank, and he wasted no time in springing to action.

At the hospital he asked the director if they had a blood bank. The answer was no. Kolff asked if they wanted him to set one up. The answer was yes.

"They gave me an automobile with a soldier in front because there were snipers," Kolff remembered, "and they gave me purchase orders so that I could go to every store in the city and buy whatever I had to. And in four days time I had a blood bank ready." Thanks to the assistance of the Dutch people, who willingly lined up to donate blood, Willem established the first blood bank in Europe, which is still in existence today.

Interestingly, Kolff credits his work with blood during transfusions and setting up the blood bank with helping

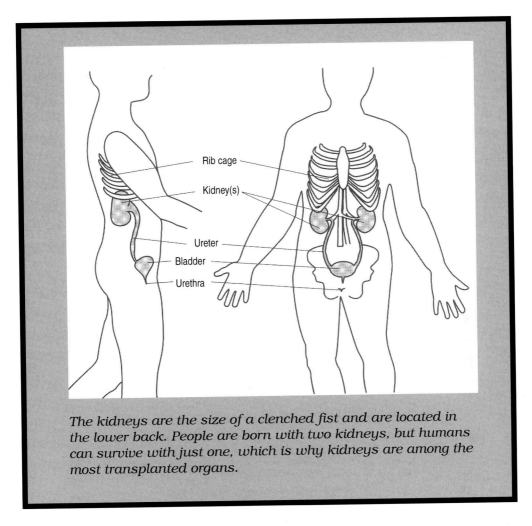

The kidneys are the size of a clenched fist and are located in the lower back. People are born with two kidneys, but humans can survive with just one, which is why kidneys are among the most transplanted organs.

him in his work with kidney patients. He said, "Having handled blood outside the body made dialysis less difficult for me."

Once he was settled in Kampen, Kolff looked forward to two things: not having to have anything to do with the Nazis, and working on developing his artificial kidney, a project he did not want the occupying Germans to know anything about. At the Kampen hospital, Willem set up his office in Room 13, which he superstitiously renumbered to be Room 12-A.

In order to create an artificial kidney, Kolff needed to understand the mechanisms by which real kidneys work and try to duplicate that through whatever material and machines he could get his hands on during wartime.

Each kidney is made up of approximately one million nephrons, which are tiny structures that produce urine as part of the process of removing wastes from the body. Each nephron contains a glomerulus, which is a network of capillaries. The glomerulus is the place where kidney filtration actually takes place. In turn, each glomerulus is attached to a renal tubule, a microscopic tube that goes to a collection area. After blood is filtered by the glomeruli, the remaining fluid travels through the tubules, where water and chemicals are either added or taken out according to the body's need at that moment. The final waste product of this process is urine, which is sent to the bladder through another tube called the ureter. The average person excretes, or gets rid of, about two quarts of urine every day.

The kidneys are remarkable, filtering about 50 gallons of fluid every 24 hours, removing toxins and keeping a person healthy. When the kidneys become damaged, either because of illness or injury, they might not be able to work properly. When that happens, waste products start to build up in the body, and it causes the person to feel sick. This is known as kidney, or renal, failure. Renal failure can be either acute or chronic.

Acute renal failure is sudden, severe damage to the kidneys or the loss of kidney function and is typically caused by severe infections, poisoning or injury. It can usually be reversed when the source of the problem is eliminated. Most doctors in the 1920s and 1930s looked to dialysis or an artificial kidney to assist people just temporarily until their kidneys recovered.

Chronic renal failure, however, is a condition that cannot be reversed or cured. It is frequently caused by a disease such as diabetes or Alport's syndrome, which afflicts children. Kolff believed the proper artificial kidney could also help these patients live longer.

Among the problems that had confounded doctors and researchers is that anytime they performed an invasive procedure—made an incision or in any way opened the body—blood clots could form. If a blood clot lodged in the brain, it would kill the patient. But by 1938, a new drug called heparin had been introduced. Heparin helped prevent clotting and gave Kolff a head start over the researchers who had tackled the problem before the drug was available.

The biggest problem in constructing the artificial kidney was finding a material that would act as a filter. Through a chance meeting, Kolff discovered just the material to use: sausage casing.

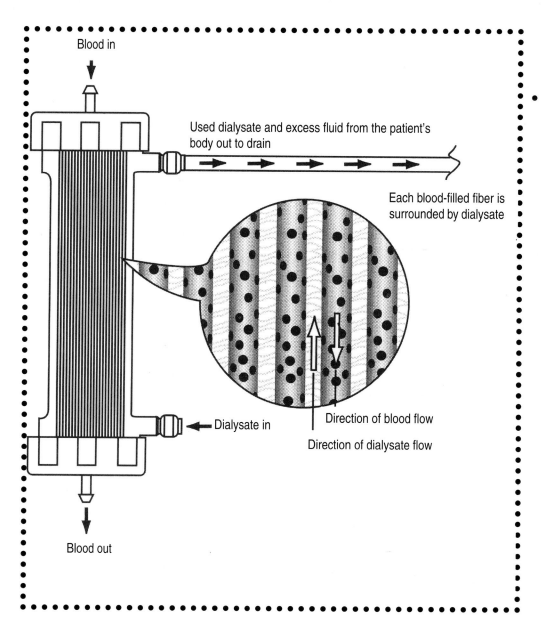

This dialysis diagram shows the direction of blood and dialysate flow, which runs in counter-current directions. As blood passes through the filter area, urea and other waste products move out of the blood and into dialysate, effectively cleaning the blood.

Chapter 4
Surgical Sausage Casing

Not long after Jan Bruning died, Kolff met with a biochemistry teacher at Groningen University named Professor Brinkman. It was Brinkman who first told Willem about the amazing properties of cellophane, which is a thin, clear, membrane-like substance that was then being used as an artificial sausage casing. Brinkman told Kolff that in experiments he had conducted, when two solutions were separated by cellophane, an exchange of molecules took place. The cellophane acted as a kind of fine mesh filter.

Because the area of greater concentration moved to the area of lower concentration, Kolff immediately realized that cellophane could be just the material for which he was searching. He wanted blood with high concentrations of urea and other wastes to pass through to an area that had none so that the waste would be filtered out of the blood. Not only that, cellophane was inexpensive and readily available.

"Cellophane tubing looks like ribbon, but it's hollow," explains Kolff. "If you have blood inside here, small molecules will go through the pores of the membrane to the outside where you have the dialyzing fluid. So urea and other products that the kidneys normally excrete will go out. And another thing happens. Sodium chloride and other electrolytes will also go out. So, you add them to the dialyzing fluid on the outside, and they go out and in, and you get an equilibration through this membrane. If the sodium is too low, it goes higher; if it's too high, it goes lower. This normalizes the electrolytes in the blood plasma."

But knowing what you want to do and getting it to work are two different things, as Willem discovered. He knew he wanted to remove urea and other products that are excreted by the kidney. What he needed to figure out was the best process to make that happen. It ended up being a case of trial and error and educated guesses.

Kolff explains his method: "Whenever I see a problem, I try to reduce it to simple terms. If the problem is very complicated, then look at whether or not there is a simple component to it. Reduce the complicated problem to something that you can understand, and that perhaps you can do something about."

Kolff filled a small piece of cellophane tubing with blood to which he had added urea and heparin, to prevent clotting. He sealed the skin at both ends, attached it to a board and manually agitated it in a saline bath. After half an hour he measured the urea and discovered it had all passed from the blood to the rinsing solution. Willem felt a surge of optimism. His artificial kidney would work. Now all he had to do was make a machine large enough to handle enough blood to help a patient.

When Kolff had first started working on his artificial kidney back at Groningen, his colleagues had responded with skepticism and, in some cases, outright ridicule. At the time, the only person who supported him completely was Professor Daniels. The first four apparatuses Willem built failed. Even so, Daniels had encouraged Kolff to pursue his idea. Now Willem felt vindicated and wished his professor were alive to share the moment. He would never forget the support the professor had given him, and that example

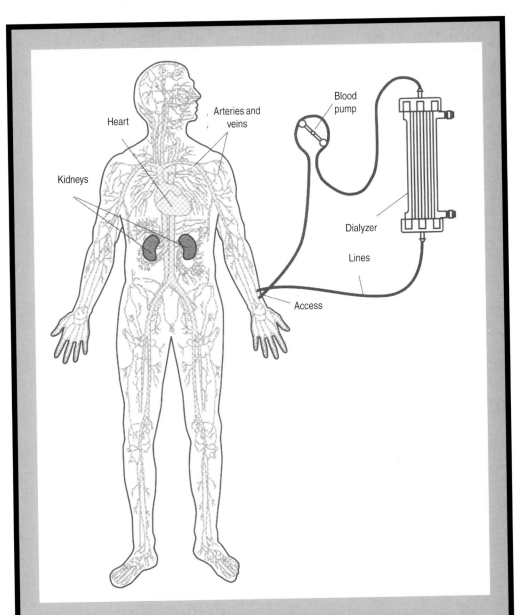

Heart

Arteries and veins

Kidneys

Blood pump

Dialyzer

Lines

Access

This figure shows the circulation in the human body. During dialysis, the blood pump acts like the human heart, pushing blood through the lines (vessels). The dialyzer, or artificial kidney, cleans the blood, which is then returned to the patient's own circulation.

would later greatly influence the way Kolff worked with young researchers.

"All my life I've tried to follow that example and, where possible, allow my students to follow their interest," Kolff would say years later. "I know where I want to get in the long run, and we don't go there in a straight line, because these students want to go this way or that way. It takes longer, but it makes their life much more interesting if they can do it their way. Eventually we'll get where we want to be."

To help build his artificial kidney, Kolff enlisted the help of Hendrik Berk, whose family owned the local enamel factory. Berk agreed to manufacture a giant horizontal rotating drum made to Kolff's precise specifications. All the while, they had to hide their activities from the occupying Germans.

The drum itself was made of varnished wood. Its lower portion rotated in an enamel tub, which contained a rinsing solution. Cellophane was wrapped around the drum in a spiral pattern.

The drum worked in a similar way to the cellophane attached to the board. When blood was put into the cellophane, it would always move to its lowest level, so as the drum turned, gravity forced the blood to work from one end of the wet cellophane to the other. Kolff had also gotten a rotating coupling, or connector, from a Ford dealer, which allowed the cellophane to be inserted through a hollow axle and remain undisturbed as the drum turned. The device was crude and primitive by today's standards, but it was about to make history.

Kolff and Berk finished construction of what would turn out to be the first clinically usable artificial kidney in 1942. In an interesting footnote, Kolff had his artificial kidney built for free. "When it came time to pay the enamel factory, it turned out that the Germans did not allow any Dutch company to work for anybody else but the German army, so the enamel factory never could give me a bill, and I never paid for it."

Now that Kolff had a working model of his artificial kidney, he needed to try it out on some patients. That would be the true test of whether his idea would work. It would be a while before he had the opportunity, because many of the people he worked with still thought he was chasing medical rainbows. Instead, he was about to find the dialysis pot of gold.

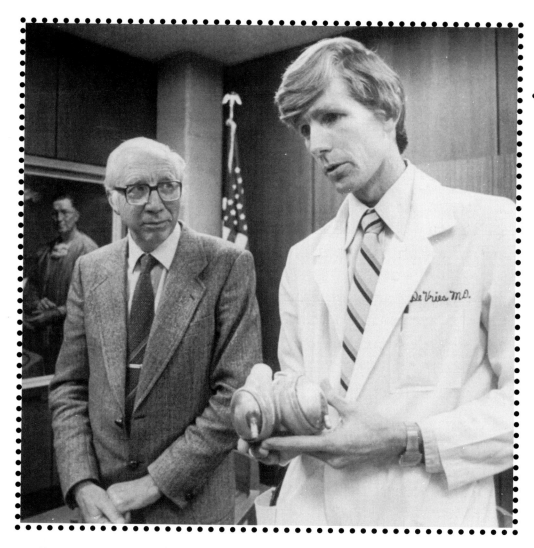

William Kolff (left) is shown here with Dr. William DeVries, the surgeon who performed the first artificial heart transplant using the Jarvik 7.

Chapter 5

Success

Kolff brought his artificial kidney home from the enamel factory and moved it into Room 12-A. To his dismay, it sat unused for a long time. None of the other doctors believed it could work and didn't refer any of their patients to him. Finally, Kolff convinced them to let him try the machine, but at first the only patients he got were those people either already in a coma or in such late stages of renal failure as to make their recovery almost impossible. But they were all Kolff had to work with when he began the first clinical trials of his invention in 1943.

He started slowly, dialyzing only a small amount of blood, then waiting a couple of days to see if the patient had any adverse reaction. When she didn't, he took more blood and continued the process. Ironically, it was the freedom of working without governmental oversight and without any attention being paid by the then established medical community that Kolff credits with his success.

"At that time if either an institutional review committee for research on human patients, or the FDA had been breathing down my neck, the artificial kidney would never have been made. Never. My conscience was my only brake. Otherwise, I could do what I wanted. But I had to explain to the patient what I was going to do, and I always did."

As he feared, the first patients he treated were too far along with their disease for the artificial kidney's dialysis to do them any good. Agonizingly for Willem, all but one of the first 15 people he treated died, although in every single case their deaths were due to complications caused by uremia and not by the artificial kidney. Kolff believed the one person who survived would have survived without his machine.

Although watching the people die was emotionally draining for Kolff, he learned a lot. The process itself appeared safe overall, but there were still several problems to solve.

Not only did Kolff need to calculate the proper composition of the dialyzing fluid so that the patient's electrolyte balance would be correct, he also needed to find an easy and safe way to connect the patient to the cellophane tube, because repeated dialysis tended to damage the veins and sometimes cause hemorrhaging. Kolff's team was able to keep one patient alive for 26 days—until his blood vessels became too damaged for further access. Plus, because heparin was so new, nobody knew for sure what the best dosage was to use. Each time Kolff used the machine he was able to improve the procedure more and more.

As time went on, Kolff saw encouraging signs that his machine was fulfilling its promise. Even in patients who died, their urea levels had dropped and some actually awoke from their comas and were able to talk. It was those small victories that kept Kolff going. He believed enough in his machine that he had eight more made and managed to smuggle them under the noses of the Germans to various cities around the Netherlands, including The Hague and Amsterdam. He also kept a machine at each local hospital so that he could perform dialysis wherever it was needed. He figured the best way to protect the machines from being destroyed by German bombs was to have them in different

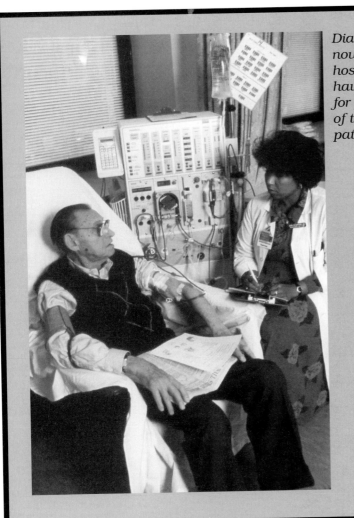

Dialysis machines are now found in every hospital. The machines have been responsible for prolonging the lives of thousands of patients each year.

places. And to prevent the Germans from taking credit for his work, he published the results of his experiments in Scandinavian medical journals.

On June 6, 1944, the allies invaded Normandy in a military offensive known as D-Day. The following month, on July 27, Kolff was forced to abandon his work on the artificial kidney: the allies were advancing on Holland, poised to destroy the German rocket installations there that had been used to bomb London. A year later, Hitler was defeated and the war was over, and the Netherlands was once again free. Eager to get back to work, on September 3, 1945, Kolff prepared to give his 17th patient dialysis. This one would survive solely as a result of Kolff's artificial kidney. The biggest irony for Willem, however, was that 67-year-old Maria Sophia Schafstadt was a prison patient, charged with collaborating with the Germans.

"Many of my fellow countrymen would have liked to wring her neck," Kolff acknowledged. "She was brought to us in acute renal failure and my duty is not to wring her neck, but to treat her."

Schafstadt was brought to the hospital near death, her condition the result of kidneys damaged by a diseased gall bladder. Kolff immediately recognized she was in the early stages of a fatal uremic coma and needed dialysis right away. However, he had to get permission first and waited impatiently until she had no visible kidney function at all: then he was given the go-ahead. For 12 hours, Kolff performed dialysis. It appeared that another patient was destined to die.

After he had dialyzed 80 liters, which is over 21 gallons, or about 14 cycles, of Schafstadt's blood, he took the patient off the artificial kidney and waited. Although her blood pressure had gone down and her urea level was reduced, Kolff was not optimistic. Still, he remained at the hospital all night, keeping vigil over the unconscious woman.

To Kolff's surprise and joy, the next morning Schafstadt came out of her coma and produced a very small quantity of urine. Kolff performed another round of dialysis. Her urea level went down as her kidneys started producing more and more urine. In less than a week, her kidneys were functioning normally. Now there was absolutely no doubt—Kolff's artificial kidney worked and could save lives. For the first time, medical science had prevailed against kidney disease.

Often, medical advances happen simultaneously because teams of doctors all over the world are working on the same problem. But in the case of the artificial kidney, Kolff was alone. When the war ended, he discovered, to his surprise, his work had not been duplicated anywhere. In 1946 he donated artificial kidneys to London, New York, and Montreal, eager to help as many people as possible. And he did so without ever patenting his invention, meaning people could make their own version of his machines without having to pay Kolff any money for it. Willem was much more interested in saving lives than in reaping personal financial rewards. That would come anyway as his machine revolutionized kidney care.

While some people might be satisfied with creating one invention that would benefit so many people, for Willem Kolff it was just the beginning. Over the next half century, he would become known as one of the greatest medical inventors and innovators of all time and earn the nickname the Father of Artificial Organs.

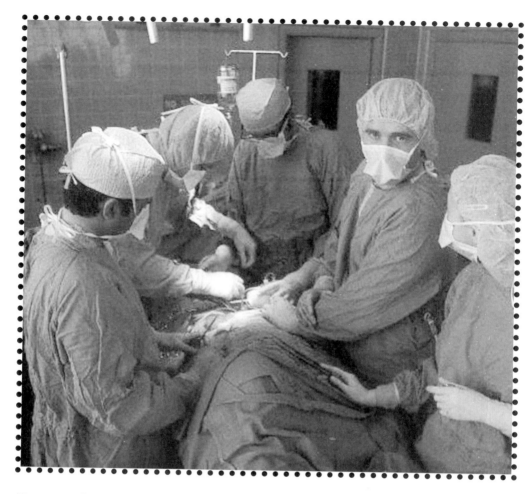

Doctors first performed transplants on animals. This photograph is from the first cow transplant.

Chapter 6

New Frontiers

● ●

In 1950, Kolff and his family left their native Holland and moved to the United States. He joined the Cleveland Clinic Foundation, where he served as scientific director of the Artificial Organs Program and worked on improving his kidney machine. But Kolff, who wasn't satisfied with resting on past successes, began working on numerous other projects, such as developing a heart-lung machine, which would help keep patients alive during open-heart surgery.

As Kolff studied the heart, he became intrigued with the idea of inventing an artificial one. In 1957 he developed the first totally artificial heart and set about doing some clinical trials with it. Although his first patient, a laboratory dog, lived for only 90 minutes, Kolff was undaunted. He spent the next 25 years working on many different models and prototypes of artificial hearts.

Kolff left Cleveland in 1967 for Utah to direct the Division of Artificial Organs and the Institute for Biomedical Engineering at the University of Utah. While there, Kolff was in charge of teams who worked to improve his previous inventions and teams who developed new ones: artificial eyes, ears and limbs. Again he made significant advances and developed devices that greatly improved the quality of life for many people.

In 1982 William DeVries implanted the Jarvik-7 artificial heart, developed by Kolff, Donald Olsen and Robert Jarvik, into a patient named Barney Clark. Clark eventually

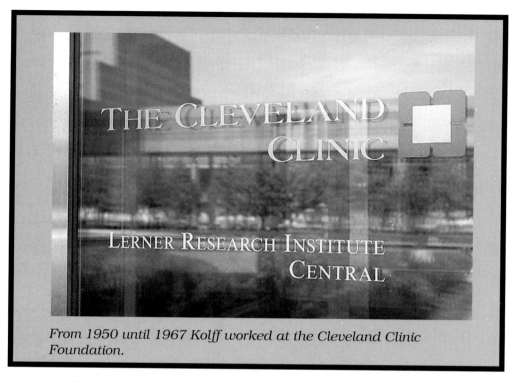

From 1950 until 1967 Kolff worked at the Cleveland Clinic Foundation.

succumbed to complications from the transplant, but the operation opened the door to the possibility of one day creating a truly portable artificial heart—a dream Kolff would continue working on the rest of his professional life.

Although Kolff officially retired in 1986, his legacy of work continues to set the standard in the field of artificial organ research. Over the course of his life he has published more than 600 articles and been honored with more than 100 professional awards. Perhaps most prestigious is that the Smithsonian Institution acquired a collection of Kolff's inventions as an example of scientific and medical research at its best.

Still, though, Kolff will always be best remembered as the doctor who first conquered the ravaging effects of kidney disease and laid the foundation for other medical advances

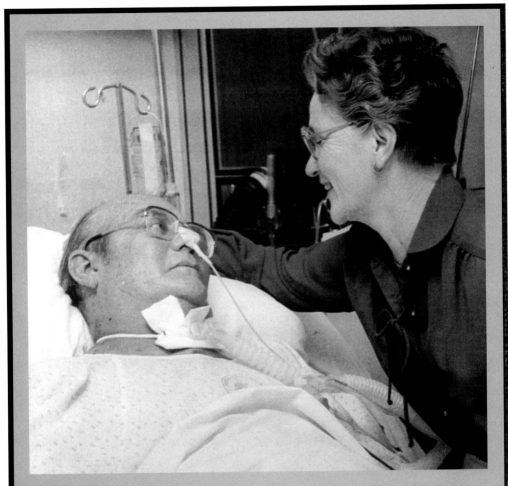

Barney Clark was the first recipient of an artificial heart. He is shown here with his wife, with whom he spent his extra days of life.

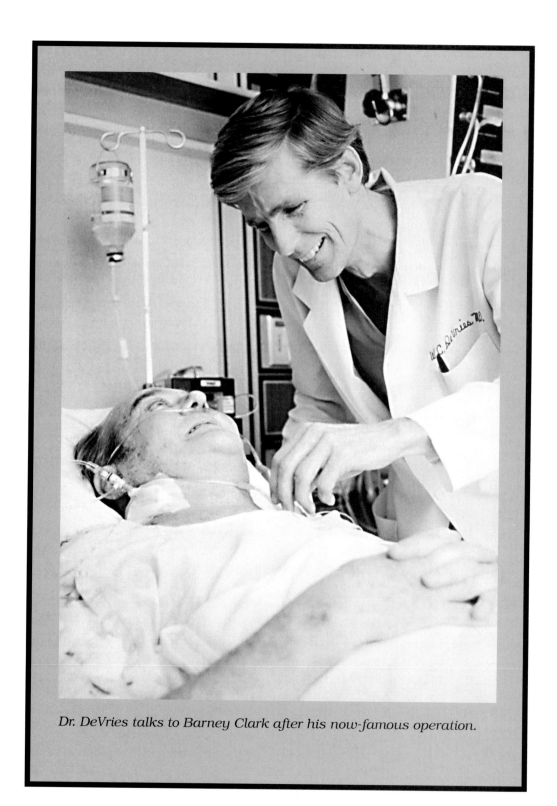

Dr. DeVries talks to Barney Clark after his now-famous operation.

in the field. Today, even people with complete kidney failure can now lead reasonably normal lives because of modern dialysis techniques and new successes in transplantation. It is estimated that dialysis keeps more than 120,000 Americans alive every year who would otherwise have died from kidney failure.

Looking back over his life's work, Kolff says one of the most important lessons he learned was to not give up. "There are a lot of people that are a great deal smarter than I am. So I have to work very hard, but I'm extremely persistent. If I cannot get there one way, I try another way.

"If I had to give any advice to younger people who want to accomplish something, first try to simplify what you want to do, and see whether or not you can do it. No reason to bump your head against the wall if you don't see a little hole in it. But if you see a possibility, then take it on. If you cannot get there one way, try another way."

Willem Kolff Chronology

1911   Born February 14 in Leyden, Netherlands

1938   Earns medical degree at University of Leyden; works at University of Groningen Hospital

1940   Participates in establishing the first operational blood bank in Europe

1942   With Berk, constructs the first clinically usable artificial kidney

1946   Receives Ph.D. from the University of Groningen

1947   Wins Amory Prize

1950   With his family, immigrates to the United States; begins association with Cleveland Clinic Foundation

1955   Produces the first clinically useful membrane oxygenator for a heart-lung machine

1956   Becomes a U.S. citizen

1957   Implants the first artificial heart in an animal

1964   Named one of the nation's top 10 physicians; awarded prestigious Cameron Prize for Practical Therapeutics by the University of Edinburgh

1965   Develops silicone rubber heart for a calf

1967   Accepts position of Director of the Division of Artificial Organs and the Institute for Biomedical Engineering at the University of Utah

1969   Honored with Valentine Medal and Award

1975   Introduces Wearable Artificial Kidney, making dialysis portable

1986   Retires from full-time research on 75th birthday but continues to work part-time

1990   Named by *Life* magazine as one of the 100 most important Americans of the 20th century

1998   The Smithsonian Institution acquires the Kolff Collection, which includes the first artificial kidney

Dialysis and Artificial Heart Timeline

1667 First blood transfusion performed by Jean-Baptiste Denis

1865 Joseph Lister perfects antiseptic surgery

1900 Austrian doctor Karl Landsteiner discovers three different blood types, A, B, and C (now called O)

1905 Alexis Carrel paves the way for future organ transplants with his techniques of rejoining severed blood vessels

1913 First practical demonstration of continuous dialysis of blood (vividiffusion) by American research team John Jacob Abel, Leonard Rowntree and J.J. Turner at Johns Hopkins Hospital in Baltimore

1924 German scientist George Haas performs dialysis on the first human patient

1932 Pacemaker invented by A. S. Hyman

1937 Pure form of heparin obtained for use in humans

1942 Kolff introduces first artificial kidney

1945 First record of patient being saved by artificial kidney

1957 Kolff tests artificial heart in animals; Earl Bakken, Robert Jarvik, and C. Walton Lillehie develop first externally worn, battery-powered pacemaker

1967 Christiaan Barnard performs world's first human heart transplant

1981 Under Kolff's supervision, Robert Jarvik designs an artificial heart intended to be used on a human

1982 William C. DeVries implants the Jarvik heart into patient Barney Clark

Further Reading

Books

Ballard, Carol. *The Heart and Circulatory System.* The Human Body. Austin, Tex.: Raintree Steck-Vaughn, 1997.

Bankston, John. *Christiaan Barnard and the Story of the First Successful Heart Transplant.* Bear, Del.: Mitchell Lane Publishers, 2002.

Bankston, John. *Robert Jarvik and the First Artificial Heart.* Bear, Del.: Mitchell Lane Publishers, 2002.

Beckelman, Laurie. *Transplants.* The Facts About Series. New York: Crestwood House, 1990.

Casanellas, Antonio, and Ali Garousi (illustrator). *Great Discoveries and Inventions That Improved Human Health.* Milwaukee: Gareth Stevens, 2000.

Dowswell, Paul. *Medicine.* Great Inventions. Portsmouth, N.H.: Heinemann Library, 2001.

Hurst, J. Willis, Stuart Hurst, Jackie Ball, Patricia J. Wynne, and Patsy Bryan (illustrator). *The Heart: The Kids' Question and Answer Book.* New York: McGraw-Hill, 1998.

Kittredge, Mary, and C. Everett Koop. *Organ Transplants.* Broomall, Penn.: Chelsea House, 1999.

Parker, Steve. *Medical Advances.* 20th Century Inventions. Austin, Tex.: Raintree Steck-Vaughn, 1998.

Web Sites

American Academy of Achievement, Hall of Science and Exploration
http://www.achievement.org/autodoc/page/kol0int-1
Kidney Dialysis Foundation
http://www.kdf.org.sg
Colorado Health Site Kidney Disease and Dialysis Center

http://www.coloradohealthsite.org/

Interview with Willem Kolff

http://www.stanford.edu/dept/HPS/transplant/html/
kolff.html

Western Skies Dialysis Education Page

http://www.westernskiesdialysis.com/education/index.html

Glossary of Terms

acute: describes a disease that happens suddenly and requires immediate attention. Acute renal failure is a condition in which the kidneys suddenly stop working.

Alport's syndrome: an inherited condition that results in kidney disease. It generally develops during early childhood and is more serious in boys than in girls. The condition can lead to end-stage renal disease, as well as to hearing and vision problems.

bladder: a balloon-shaped organ inside the pelvis that holds urine.

blood vessels: the veins, arteries and capillaries through which blood flows.

capillaries: extremely small blood vessels with walls only one cell thick. These walls allow the exchange of oxygen, carbon dioxide, salts, and other vital nutrients and waste products between the blood and the body's organs.

chronic: lasting a long time. Chronic diseases develop slowly. Chronic renal failure may develop over many years and lead to end-stage renal disease.

dialysate: a cleansing solution of water and chemicals used in dialysis.

dialysis: the separation of waste matter from the blood using either a machine or other methods.

dialyzer: a part of the hemodialysis machine. The dialyzer has two sections separated by a membrane; one section holds dialysate, the other holds the patient's blood.

dyslexia: a learning disability that makes it difficult to read.

edema: swelling caused by too much fluid in the body.

electrolytes: chemicals such as sodium, potassium, magnesium, and chloride found in body fluids that result from the breakdown of salts. The kidneys control the amount of electrolytes in the body, so when the kidneys fail, electrolytes get out of balance, causing potentially serious health problems. Dialysis can correct this imbalance.

end-stage renal disease: kidney failure that requires dialysis or a kidney transplant.

excrete: to get rid of metabolic waste materials from an individual cell or an entire body.

glomerulonephritis: a condition in which the capillaries in the kidney are inflamed.

glomerulus: a network of capillaries on a kidney nephron that is the site of kidney filtration.

hemodialysis: purification of blood by dialysis; the use of a machine to clean wastes from the blood after the kidneys have failed.

heparin: a substance made by the liver that helps prevent blood from clotting. A pure form is now used as a blood thinner and to prevent clotting during dialysis.

hormone: a natural chemical produced in one part of the body and released into the blood to trigger or regulate particular functions of the body.

hypertension: higher-than-normal blood pressure.

internist: a kind of doctor who specializes in internal medicine and is expert at diagnosing diseases.

kidneys: the two bean-shaped organs located near the middle of the back that filter wastes from the blood and excretes them as urine.

nephrons: tiny structures in the kidneys that produce urine during the process of removing wastes from the body; each kidney is made up of about one million nephrons.

renal: having to do with the kidneys.

renal tubule: part of a nephron of the kidney consisting of a microscopic tube extending from the glomerulus to a collecting duct. The functions of reabsorption and secretion occur across its walls.

summa cum laude: with highest praise.

toxic: poisonous.

transfusion: a transfer of blood from one person to another.

transplant: to transfer an organ from one person to another.

urea: an end product of protein metabolism and the main compound of urine.

uremia: a toxic condition resulting from kidney disease in which waste products normally filtered out by the kidneys build up in the bloodstream.

ureter: one of two narrow tubes that carry urine from the kidneys to the bladder.

urine: the liquid produced by the kidneys; it carries wastes from the body, including water, salts, ammonia, urea, and urochrome, which gives urine its color.

Index